The 16 Hour Diet

By

Ashley Barnes

Copyright © 2014 by Ashley Barnes. All rights reserved. Except as permitted under the U.S. Copyright Act of 1976, no part of this publication may be reproduced, distributed, or transmitted in any form or by any means, or stored in a database or retrieval system, without the prior and express written permission of the publisher

Disclaimer

The information in this book is based on how I lost weight. The information in this plan is based on my own personal experience and my own interpretations of available research. This is not medical advice and I am not a medical doctor. You should consult with your physician to make sure this diet plan is appropriate for your individual circumstance. If you have any health issues or concerns, please consult with your physician. Always consult your physician before beginning or making any changes in your diet or exercise program. For diagnosis and treatment of illness and injuries, and for advice regarding medications, consult your Doctor. If you are pregnant or breastfeeding, consult with your doctor before beginning this diet.

"Don't spend the rest of your life wondering if you can do it. START NOW."

I would like to give thanks to God for the opportunity to write this book, and to help others. I would also like to thank my husband and family for supporting me and helping me achieve this goal. I hope you enjoy reading this book as much as I enjoyed writing it.

Table of contents

- About me 6
- Intro..12
- What's your Why......................15
- Let's Get Started......................20
- The 16 Hour Diet.....................24
- Why this works........................38
- Health Benefits of The 16 Hour Diet..49
- Turbo Charge!!!......................61
- Ready set go 78
- Frequently Asked Questions................................96
- Bonus recipes 107

"I will fight for it! I will not give up! I will reach my goal and absolutely NOTHING will stop me!"

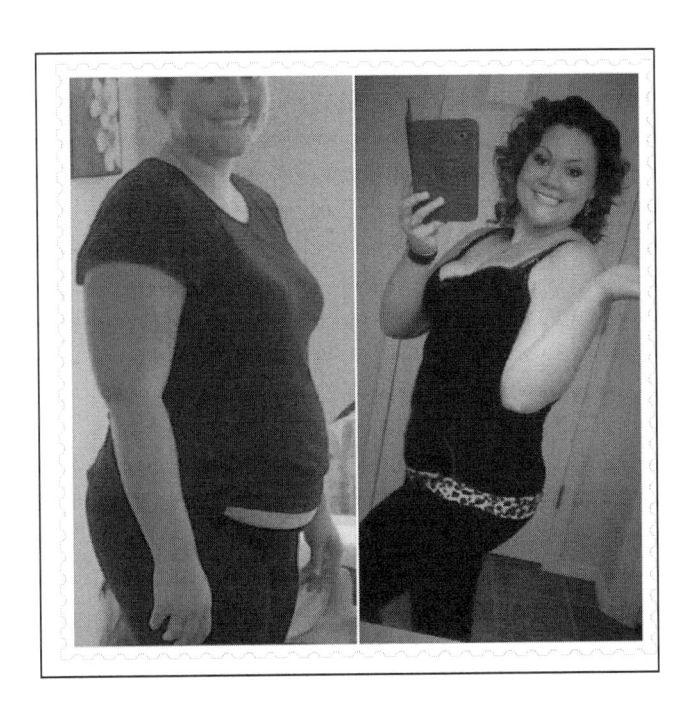

About me

My name is Ashley and I'm a mother of 4 beautiful children and married to my best friend and husband, Chris. I am also a

Certified Life Coach specializing in health and fitness. I have a deep passion for helping others with all aspects of life, but it didn't take long to discover that weight loss is especially important to me. Due to my own journey and struggles with losing weight, I was already putting some of my time to researching how to lose weight the best way. After I started helping others in their weight loss journey, I realized just how important this is to so many people. The struggles and triumphs of others is eventually what compelled me to dedicate my coaching to helping people lose weight. This also helped me in my own journey.

My struggles with losing weight started after I had my first child, and continued with each pregnancy. For each of my four children, I've gained an average of 80 pounds. Of course, this was not fun for me, so I tried to lose the weight each time. I would go from diet to diet, fad to fad, product to product, so trust me when I say I've tried everything under the sun. I've given honest tries to every restrictive diet, or intense workout programs, and have spent many late night hours watching those infomercials trying to find the newest thing. I could write a whole book on the things I've tried, and I would need my entire book proceeds to cover the many dollars wasted.

I will say that I wasn't completely unsuccessful in my attempts to lose weight. If you want something bad enough, and work hard, you will get there. With my first two children, I was able to lose the pregnancy weight, eighty pounds each time. That is a great thing, and I felt really accomplished, but I wasn't happy, and I couldn't afford the time, money and effort these methods required to maintain, let alone, continue to move down towards my ideal weight. You can only go so long with a restrictive 1200 calorie diet, and your toddlers don't really understand why Mommy has to work out for three hours every day, instead of playing with them. It was these reasons that led me to continue to research and find a way to effectively lose weight, yet live my life as a full time Mom.

After my third child, I started looking into bodybuilding forums and websites, mainly for my husband, who was trying to build muscle. I stumbled across fasting, and more specifically, intermittent fasting. Many bodybuilders were using fasting during their cutting phase, when they lose excess fat and prepare for competitions. Now I wasn't getting ready to 'compete', and I wasn't aiming to bulk my bicep's, but the way they lost weight so easily intrigued me. I also didn't like the idea of fasting, because when you're a full time Mom, it isn't something you really consider. Yet, I continued to research and learn more about intermittent fasting, or fasting. My husband and I decided to give it a try, and that's when The 16 Hour Diet was born.

I was eventually able to lose the pregnancy weight from my third baby, and continue to lose weight, without drastically changing my diet, and without taking time away from my family. The first month I lost 12 pounds. I was shocked at what was happening to me. I didn't use expensive meal plans with ingredients that Wal-Mart doesn't even carry and my husband's favorite thing was I didn't waste any more money giving '4 easy payments' of whatever for the newest workout program. I lost weight in a healthy manner and it was amazing. I turned my body in to a fat burning machine. I lost 68 pounds in about 6 months. Yes you just read that correctly that was 68 pounds gone. I knew this was it. I wanted to share with every single person that was struggling to lose weight. So I started writing this guide book. As I write this, I'm recovering from my fourth cesarean for our newest addition, and I'm already losing weight. It's now time for me to help others do the same, by sharing The 16

Hour Diet with everyone. I am losing weight right now with The 16 Hour Diet and I couldn't wait any longer to share my secret. Join me in losing weight and becoming healthy. I hope you enjoy this guide, and more importantly, I hope it helps you lose weight like it did for me before and is doing for me now. Get ready to commit yourself and watch your body change.

"Every Accomplishment starts with the decision to try."

<u>Intro</u>

    Thank you for reading The 16 Hour Diet, and congratulations for taking a step to a healthier you. I am so excited to share my experiences with you, and hopefully save you from the pain, stress, and cost that I spent trying to lose weight. This book is basically a collection of my thoughts, ideas, and interpretations of losing weight with Intermittent Fasting. If you follow this guide, you will turn your body in to a fat burning machine and feel better, look better, and be healthier overall. Gosh I am Excited about this I know this can change your life because it helped me and is helping me change mine.

The 16 Hour Diet is an extension on fasting, and more specifically, Intermittent Fasting. I found that those body builders were actually keeping a very big secret, one that is extremely effective in losing weight. It's not just the body builders though, because people in general have been fasting in one way or another, for generations. Now, I don't propose you go days without food, so don't worry. That's the great thing about Intermittent Fasting. The definition of Intermittent Fasting is alternating cycles of eating and not eating. Basically, you eat for a period of time, and then you don't eat for a period of time.

Now, it's not as simple as this or my book would only need to be a paragraph, but The 16 Hour Diet is founded on this simple principle, and below are my interpretations and recommendations on how to use Intermittent Fasting to lose weight. It doesn't matter who you are or what you weigh. The most important part is that this method is easy, really easy, and this book is everything you need to get started. Are you ready to change your body, make your body work for you, and lose weight quickly and easily?

"Put ALL your excuses aside and remember this; You are capable!"

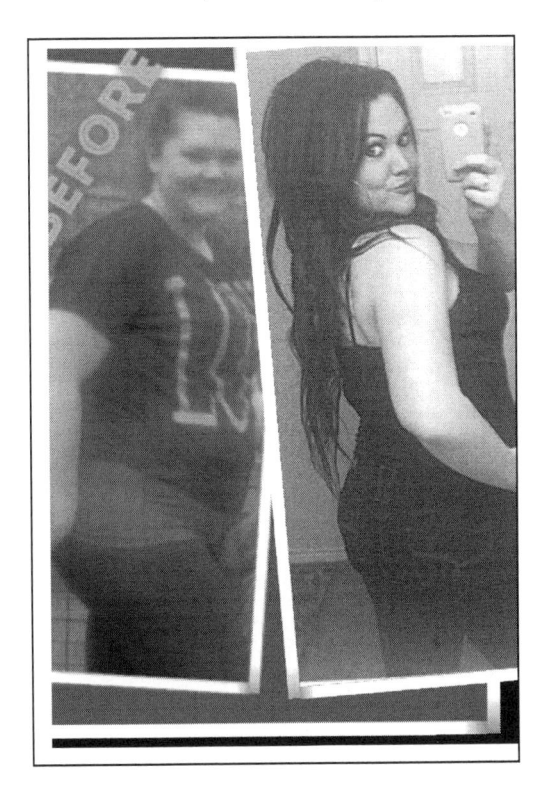

What is your Why?

Why do you want to lose weight? This is the most important section, and the most important question in this book. Even outside of this book, I would still say this question is the key to losing weight. Now when I ask for your 'Why', I mean it. Why do you want to lose weight? Take some time right now and ask yourself this...I can wait....Okay. Seriously, have you asked yourself why you want to lose weight? Have you pondered why you spend so much time, effort and money to lose weight? I mean, why are you even reading this book? There has to be a reason, something that makes you do these things, and it's important to know what that reason is, and always keep it in front of you. This 'Why' is the thing that will keep you going when times get hard, and motivate you when you feel like quitting. Find your why, and you'll find the key to your success.

I have my Why's around me at all times because I'm still on my journey of weight loss. My first Why has to do with my family history. My father passed away at the young age of 58 due to Obesity and the health problems obesity can cause. When my father passed away, that was a slap in my face. Mainly because he was always a 'big' guy and it was normal to see him that size. I had even become overweight as a young adult, but it wasn't seen as an issue because of my family and their body types. Yet, when he died, and why he died, it made me stop and take a good hard look at my own life. I realized then that, if I live a similar lifestyle to my dad, I could share in his early fate. I knew then that wasn't an option, because I knew how it felt to lose a parent at a young age, and I didn't want that for my children. That's when I found my first why.

It was after I had my second child that I discovered another Why. Due to multiple cesarean section operations, large weight gains with each pregnancy, and osteoarthritis in my knees and hips from past medical issues, I wasn't able to move and play with my kids in the backyard like I wanted. I knew I couldn't reverse the arthritis or past surgeries, and I couldn't undo the cesarean, but I could change something that could help alleviate the pain and difficulties those things caused. If I could lose enough weight, my quality of life would improve. This was also validated by my doctor and OB/GYN. If I could lose weight, I would feel like myself, and not like some statue that couldn't move and go when I wanted.

My third why comes simply from every time I've gone to a department store and had to go straight to the 'larger' section! I was tired of flipping frantically through each shirt, trying to find the needle in the haystack that actually would fit. I was tired of seeing girl's with super cute clothes and styles, and then not being able to find the same things. Don't even mention clearance racks, because those were practically off limits to a person my size. I wanted to be able to wear the cute styles, look hot, and feel great, instead of feeling anything less. When I sat back and thought it through, I had three reasons to drive me to lose weight. I wanted to look great, feel great, and most importantly, have great health.

Now that I've given my Why's, I want for you to think about why you really want to lose weight. Is it because you want to fit that hot little bikini before summer, or is it because you want to add years to your life and live for your kids and family? Whatever your reasons, keep it, meditate on it, pray on it, write it down right here, and you could even post it online. Every time you feel like quitting, or are tempted to break The 16 Hour Diet, come back to your Why and remember what you're doing this for. Below I have created a space for you to write down your why. Take a moment before we move forward to write your why down.

_____

_____

_____

"1 pound of fat is 3,500 calories. If you want to lose 1 lb. per week, then just burn 500 calories per day more than you eat or minus those calories. Weight loss is science, not magic."

Let's Get Started

It's important to clarify that The 16 Hour Diet is not a diet at all. It's really more of a schedule for eating. Put simply, The 16 Hour Diet tells you when to eat and when not to eat. This means that we will focus on when you eat, more than what you eat, which is counter to every other diet you've probably come across.

Of course, The 16 Hour Diet will work if you're eating clean and unprocessed foods that are high protein and low fat. But if you're like me, eating diet foods and restricting yourself from the foods you love only leads you to quitting or not being able to maintain that route. From there, you fall right back to square one, still overweight and angry and upset your efforts didn't work. I feel like this is why so many people fail their diets and don't lose weight. It's not realistic to drink a shake every day, eat minimal calories, or eat Kale and brown rice all day long. The 16 Hour Diet will put an end to that cycle right now, by allowing you to eat what you love, and still burn crazy fat!

I have found that, if you want to create healthy habits that you actually keep, then you need to start as small as possible. One day and one smart choice at a time until you reach your ultimate goal. Don't forget to use your 'Why' when you need some encouragement or refocusing. So instead of getting pumped up and trying to change everything right away, like moving to a no carb diet, or committing to a 2 hour workout program, or doing both at the same time, The

16 Hour Diet allows you to start small, and focus on one day at a time. One day at a time, and one smart choice at a time, and eventually you will change your habits, and your life. All while still losing weight. It's so simple to do this, I just want to stand on a mountain and scream it to the world!

Anyone that's ever struggled with weight loss can use The 16 Hour Diet to change their life and turn their body into a fat burning machine. Did I mention, you can still eat what you want, and you don't have to buy any workout equipment, go to any meetings, or restrict your calories so immensely that your starving and wishing you had 10 burgers in front of you. I feel that not having to tell yourself you can't have the food you want while doing The 16 Hour Diet, keeps you from feeling deprived. Eventually with this diet, you will start to crave those unhealthy things less and less. There is some scientific reason why this happens, and we'll cover that later. Right now, just know that eventually you will reach a point where you don't crave cookies and cakes all day long. So are you ready? Let's get started! Below I want you to wright down your starting weight.

 Tip: make sure you weigh in at the same time of day and also I prefer to weigh in during the morning hours. Remember that the clothes your wear can add, which is why I weigh in the mornings before I get dressed for the day.

Today on _____ I weighed in at _____.

My goal is to reach_____ weight. I can do it because I Know my why and I am worth it. Yes YOU are worth it. You can do this.

"Don't wait until you've reached your goal to be proud of yourself. Be proud of every step you take toward reaching your goal."

The 16 Hour Diet

First, I'll go over exactly when you should and shouldn't eat, and later I'll explain exactly why you do this and how it turns your body into a fat blaster.

The 16 Hour Diet is based on principles from Intermittent Fasting and how it's worked so effortlessly for me. This means we need to focus on when you are eating and when you are not eating. The goal of this diet is right there in the title, 16 hours. Therefore, your goal will be to eat for 8 hours of the day, and then go on a 16 hour diet of not eating. Sounds simple right? Let's review in detail.

In a normal day, you would wake up around 7am and get a cup of coffee with sugar and cream to wake up. If you're like me you're picking at a muffin or something your kids left out. Then after getting dressed for the day, you would grab a bite to eat for breakfast and a high calorie drink. Maybe you're the type that grabs a breakfast bar on the way out of the door, or maybe you bust out the eggs, bacon and biscuits. Mid-afternoon snack before lunch. After that you would grab lunch around noon, Oh wait its snack time again and then get home and start on dinner. After dinner, and after putting the kids to bed, maybe you would grab a snack while you read a book or watch television. That is the prototypical day for many Americans. Forget of all of that!

In order to not eat for 16 hours straight, you need to basically choose a meal, either breakfast or dinner that you will skip. For the purpose of this diet, and based on my experience, I recommend skipping breakfast, but the choice is yours. Don't let the 16 hour scare you. Most of the time is spent while you're sleeping. Basically, you're skipping breakfast and having an early dinner. Even if you're not doing The 16 Hour Diet you should always try to avoid late night snacking and eating 4 hours before bedtime. So let's assume you choose to skip breakfast and run through the same example day.

You will wake up around 7am, and instead of grabbing a cup of coffee with sugar and cream you will have coffee with a zero calorie sweetener. Or you will grab a zero calorie drink like black coffee or tea. I'll provide some examples of zero calorie drinks to use while fasting, but a few examples are water, tea or diet soda if you're looking for that caffeine boost. Then after getting dressed, you will not reach for a breakfast bar, or bust out the eggs and bacon. Instead, you will skip breakfast altogether and go on with the start of your day. Then, depending on when you ate dinner the previous day, you will eat your lunch. This means that, if you ate dinner yesterday at 7pm, you can eat your lunch for the next day at 11am. When you eat lunch, your 16 Hour Diet will effectively be over and done.

Congratulations! You finally completed a diet all the way! Seriously though, The 16 Hour Diet for that day is done, and starting at 11am, you can eat as you normally would. Once you get to dinner, get ready, because after dinner ends, which should be about 7pm for that day, you will be done eating and your next 16 Hour Diet will begin. From that point, you will not eat food, or consume calories until the next day, when you end your diet around 11am. This allows your body to stop burning energy from food all day and instead tap in to fat stores. We'll cover this in more detail soon and it's the most exciting part.

So let's recap with an overview. You stop eating on day one at 7pm. From that point on, you don't consume a calorie, not a single calorie, or a calorie filled drink until the next day when you eat lunch at 11am. However you can drink water and other Zero calorie drinks. Don't forget, this includes skipping breakfast. The majority of your 16 hours was when you were sleeping, making this an effortless diet. When you eat lunch at 11am, the diet is over, and you eat. You can chose to have lunch and dinner or you can graze thorough your 8 hours. Yes you will have Eight hours a full Eight hours to eat. So eat as you wish during your 8 hours of course you will be making better choices as you go. After dinner ends at 7pm, your next 16 Hour Diet begins. That's it! You just focus on this cycle, or really just these two times of the day. At 11am, you can start eating, and at 7pm you stop eating.

Eight hours of eating normally, including all the foods you love, and then 16 Hours of dieting, where you don't consume a single calorie. Only Water and other zero calorie drinks.

Now I've given the times of 11am and 7pm because that generally conforms to the average person's daily schedule most people can have a lunch break at 11am, and most people can commit to finishing dinner by 7pm. But, the great thing about The 16 Hour Diet is that you don't need to stick to this fixed schedule. As long as you go at least 16 hours straight of not eating or consuming calories, you can fit the times to your schedule or lifestyle. If you can't eat lunch until 12 or 1pm, then do that. Then you can finish your dinner by 8 or 9pm, depending on when you started. If you work night shift, then adjust the times to fit your schedule. That's the beauty of The 16 Hour Diet. You can also be flexible from day to day.

Let's dig a little deeper into when you should actually eat. Even though you can adjust the times to fit your schedule, keep some things in mind. You don't want to eat a meal too closely to bedtime. So if you go to bed at 10pm, I wouldn't recommend finishing you're eating at 8pm. You should finish your eating a few hours before you go to bed. This will help you sleep better, and will also improve your weight loss results. Also, you can fast or diet longer or shorter than 16 hours while you adjust to this. Through my experience, I've found that 16 hours of fasting gives the best results for weight loss without having to abstain from eating for too long. However, if you want to start with a 12 or 14 hour diet and then work your way up, then do it. Eventually, your goal should be to reach 16 hours as soon as possible to ensure you are losing weight effectively.

Also, if you feel you can go longer than 16 hours of fasting each day, then do it. This will only turbo charge your weight loss results even more. We dive deeper into Turbo Charging your weight loss in a later section and this topic is included. Lastly, you don't need to follow the same exact schedule from day to day. If you eat dinner late one day around 8pm, then simply move your lunch time for the next day to 12pm. Or if you want to fast for 18 hours one day, and then 14 the next, then do it. Overall, if you are consistent with reaching your 16 hours, you will see better results.

But the most important part of The 16 Hour Diet is to make this diet fit your lifestyle or schedule. You shouldn't feel restricted and feel like eating at your specific times is inconvenient. It should really feel like you wake up, skip breakfast, and then eat lunch and dinner as normal. Sounds easy right? Well that's because it is very easy and so much better than killing yourself over every choice you make thought the day. Now you're ready to find out the best parts about The 16 Hour Diet.

"Giving up on your goal because of one setback is like slashing your other three tires because you got one flat."

What to Eat

So, the best part about The 16 Hour Diet is that you don't need to follow a restrictive or super complicated diet of egg whites and boiled goose. Sure, if you eat clean and healthy, you will see results. That's just the simple truth of things. In the Turbo Charge section of this book, we'll cover how to pair healthy eating with The 16 Hour Diet to boost your weight loss results and burn fat faster. But for now, forget about that.

The 16 Hour Diet focuses more on when you eat by stopping you from eating during your 16 hour diet. When the 16 hours end, and it's time to eat for eight hours, the best thing to do is to resume your normal daily routine for eating. If you normally had a sandwich and a bag a chips for lunch, then have that. If you normally eat an extra-large Number #1 from your local fast food joint, then you might want to find a healthier alternative. Processed food is bad regardless of when or how you eat it, but fast food every now and then, especially when proportioned or in moderation, can be great when you're in a hurry and need something quick.

Technically, there is no magic number of calories we should all eat each day to lose weight. While most people can lose weight eating around 1,500 calories, you can assess your own personal caloric needs with a little math. Although I haven't spent much time counting calories while using The 16 Hour Diet because I haven't needed to, it's still important to understand how weight loss works at a basic level. As a rule of thumb, you never want to exceed a deficit (or eat less than) 1000 calories lower than the amount of calories you burn. The absolute minimum calorie intake should be 1200 for women and 1500 for men.

Just remember that the body works around your base metabolic rate, meaning you need a certain number of calories to maintain your current weight. This means that if you eat less than this number, you will lose weight, but if you eat more than this set number, you will gain weight. The good news is that, for most people, this number is actually pretty high, high enough to still enjoy your favorite foods. Even better is that you can change this number by building lean muscle mass and exercising regularly. To get an idea on what your metabolic caloric maintenance is, you can search "caloric maintenance calculator" online. You can also use my formula located below to find out your caloric intake number. Once you have your magic number, you can focus on eating less than this number by 500-700 calories to lose weight in a healthy way.

By skipping breakfast, you are already cutting out these calories without any effort.

Plan your meals based on a calorie deficit the day before. In order to do that, you will need to know how many calories you can consume tomorrow in order to create a deficit of at least 500 calories. Now, if you create a daily deficit of 500 calories per day, you're going to lose a minimum of a pound per week. If you create a deficit of 1000 calories per day, you will lose a minimum of two pounds per week. Each pound of fat is approximately 3500 calories, so you can pick your weight loss goal and then plan how many pounds you want to lose each week to reach that goal. Now, the only way to create that deficit is to truly know how many calories you burn, which boils down to simply knowing your numbers! Also, if you're consuming lots of sugary drinks, you should work on decreasing the amount you drink. It's better to eat your calories than to drink them. I know it's hard to drop the sodas but you can reduce them slowly and make the switch to diet.

Don't forget, during your fast you'll want to drink plenty of water. Squeeze some Zero calorie sweetener into your water to help get rid of any cravings you experience if you enjoy flavored water. You can also drink coffee, tea, or other calorie free beverages. The caffeine in coffee and tea may actually make your 16 hours a little easier to fast, since caffeine has been found to help reduce appetite cravings. I know it helps me. I personally gave up soda many years ago but I now enjoy diet coke. Remember those little steps to a healthier you this was one of mine. So yes you can have diet sodas during your 16 hours. You can also add any zero calorie sweeteners to your drinks. After a few weeks you will find that The 16 Hour Diet keeps you from craving sugar entirely. I know scary right? A day when you don't want a cookie, could that be true?

You can do it because you're worth it! At the end of the day, remember this simply formula; **Weight loss = Calories you eat – Calories you burn**

Women:

655 + (4.3 X weight in pounds) + (4.7 X height in inches) – (4.7 X age in years) = Your caloric maintenance need

Men:

66 + (6.3 X weight in pounds) + (12.9 X height in inches) – (6.8 X age in years) = Your caloric maintenance need

Now minus you deficit target from this number and write your magic number for losing weight below?

_____

"Get Focused get Fit one day one pound at a time!"

<u>Why this works</u>

So now that you know what to do, let's talk about why The 16 Hour Diet works, and how you actually lose weight with it. To understand the diet, and fasting in general, you need to understand some basic facts about metabolism.

The common myth right now in weight loss is that you need to eat 4-6 small meals a day, which speeds up your metabolism so you can burn calories. There's actually no scientific proof that supports this claim, yet there is quite a lot of proof to support the exact opposite. For example, studies have shown that it takes your body between 8 and 12 hours to burn through the food you eat in a given day. This food is stored in your body in glycogen stores, which your body converts into energy on an as needed basis. If you constantly eat food, you are constantly replenishing those glycogen stores, so your body always has a sufficient storage of energy. The problem with this is that, if you don't burn through all that you've stored in a day, the rest is saved as,

…………………………..you guessed it, FAT. If you're constantly using energy from your food stores, you never get to a point where you're using stored fat as energy. Over time you're saving fat and not burning it, simply because you don't give your body time to burn through the energy you eat daily.

The beauty of The 16 Hour Diet is that, by not eating for 16 straight hours, you allow your body to completely burn off the food you ate from the previous day, and you give it time to start grabbing its needed energy from stored fat, turning your body in to a Fat Burning Machine! Fat contains the same type of energy as food that you eat, but just in a different format. When the body depletes its glycogen stores, it takes the fat cells and converts that into useable energy, which eliminates the fat in your body. Over time, you will burn fat off your body just by allowing your body time to get to that point of using stored fat for energy.

The length of time it takes on average to deplete your glycogen stores is 8 to 12 hours. By this point, you have burned through all the food you ate, so anything past this point, you're burning strictly energy from fat cells. That's why it's better to fast for as long as you can, or at least 16 hours. For example, if you only eat during the hours of 11am and 7pm, and then you don't eat again until the next day at 11am, you will effectively be burning pure fat by the time you eat the next day. Essentially, you're ending dinner early and skipping breakfast and making lunch your first meal of the day instead. This equates to a daily 16 hour diet, which is twice the minimum time required to deplete your glycogen stores and start shifting into fat burning mode.

In addition to simply burning through your glycogen stores and tapping into your stored fat, The 16 Hour Diet works in a few more ways to help turn your body into a fat burning furnace.

1. Your body increases production of Hormones and Enzymes for burning Fat
By not eating for a long period of time, your body actually starts to produce more Growth Hormone, also known as HGH. Hormones are one key driver to your overall metabolism, so naturally if you increase these hormones, your metabolism becomes more effective in burning fat. The higher the metabolism, the

more energy your body uses while at rest and during your normal day. HGH is one of the most important hormones for burning fat because it helps transfer energy into use for building lean muscle.

Hormones would be useless without their enzyme counterparts to help them. The enzyme is responsible for releasing fat from your fat cells to then be converted into energy by the hormones. Fasting will increase enzymes such as adipose tissue hormone Sensitive Lipase that helps release fat for use. On top of that, muscle tissue Lipoprotein Lipase enzymes, also known as LPL increase. These LPL enzymes help in allowing your muscles to absorb fat as energy to be used as fuel for exercising or in your normal day. By not eating for at least 12 hours, your body starts kicking these hormones and enzymes into hyper production and your body becomes a symphony of fat burning beauty.

2. Burn your "stubborn" fat more easily

By not eating for at least 16 Hours, your body can more easily burn fat from those "stubborn" areas such as your hips and lower stomach. This happens for a few reasons. One is, as I mention above, the enzymes and hormones that burn fat are kicked into overdrive, so your body starts grabbing fat from anywhere, including stubborn areas, to burn for energy. But in addition to that, your body activates specific B2 receptors, and then shuts down A2 receptors. This happens because your body will increase the levels of catecholamine. Catecholamine will assist in stopping the A2 receptors within the fat cells of your body.

You will also increase your abdominal subcutaneous blood flow, which is basically a highway for catecholamine's to travel on. The more blood flow, the bigger the highway, which means the CCLs will be able to reach further into your fat than normal. This, paired with lower insulin levels which we'll cover in the next section, help to shut down the A2's and activate the B2's. These B2 receptors help to move the fat cells into position for your enzymes and hormones to do their work. The longer your body stays in this state, the more stored fat is moved and converted into energy. The optimum level to achieve this state is between 12-18 hours in a normal adult, which is why The 16 Hour Diet is the perfect balance. In summary, you are increasing blood flow to your stubborn fat areas, which in turns activates the right receptors while shutting off the bad receptors, in order to allow that '"stubborn" fat to be moved and used as energy and burned off.

3. You can burn more calories through the day, without working out more

Since fasting increases your metabolism, and other things such as adrenaline, your body will naturally burn more calories through the day. Weight loss breaks down into a simple formula of calories in versus calories out, so the more calories you burn during the day, the more weight you will lose. That's not it. Since your body gets to a point of releasing fat cells into energy, your body actually gains access to more energy than it normally would have. Your body fat can store hundreds of thousands of calories in fat cells, which is far more than you could ever eat in a day.

This means you will feel more energized simply because you have more access to energy for your body. When I started The 16 Hour Diet, I expected to feel bummed out, weak, slow and tired from not eating for a long time. However, I had a natural energy boost and I felt great during the times I wasn't eating, and just all through the day. This also helps me feel better about exercising and being more active, which in turn burns even more calories for weight loss and makes me want to work out more.

4. Burn Fat Instead of Sugar
Let's set the record straight right now. That sugary soda you drink in the afternoon gives you a slight boost of energy and you may feel slightly better and more energized after drinking it. This is because sugar is a form of energy for our bodies. However, it's not the best form, not even close. Our fat cells are

basically a stored form of pure energy, that when converted, can fuel our bodies for much longer than sugar can. It's kind of like a fire in the fire place. You can add some newspaper into the fire and for a few seconds, the heat and brightness of the fire increases a lot, but after that, your fire is often weaker than before. This is because that newspaper is highly combustible so it can be converted into energy very easily, but it's empty so it runs out very quickly.

Now, if you put a thick log of cedar wood in the fireplace, it will take a few minutes to catch, but once it catches, it will burn steadily and consistently for hours. This is because, while the cedar wood is harder to start, it contains much more fuel for a fire so the fire lasts longer. This is exactly like your body. Sugar is like newspaper, and fat is like the wood.

Now let's relate this to our diet. The 16 Hour Diet trains your body to burn fat cells and not sugar because your depleting all sugar and food stores by not eating, and then increasing the enzymes and hormones in your body that help tap into the fat cells. This conversion from burning sugar to burning stored fat helps you feel more energized throughout your day, and helps you lose weight easier. You'll be an actual fat burning furnace when you're all done, just like I've been saying.

5. Improve your attitude about food and improve your self-confidence

Each time you go 16 hours without eating, you are completing a diet. Congratulations! I had never ever completed any diet before this one, and when I did complete this, I felt great. There's something about setting a goal and achieving it that makes you feel good about yourself. Each 16 diet is basically a small goal towards your one big goal along the way. Each time you reach a small goal, you feel more motivated for the next and eventually reach your big goal over time. Most productivity experts will tell you to set your big goal first but then set a bunch of small goals that get you there. This is exactly how The 16 Hour Diet works. You set a goal each day to not eat anything until the next day, and when you make it to that point, you feel great about achieving your goal. This positive reinforcement continues to build until you feel completely empowered over your food choices and your body, and ultimately, I think that's what we all want.

6. Eat all the foods you love without feeling Guilty

I saved this one for last because it's my favorite. By not eating for 16 Hours, when it is actually time for you to eat, you can eat the foods you love without feeling guilty. This is because you are already in a caloric deficit, meaning you have burned more calories than you consume. Plus, your body is working in overdrive to burn stored fat, so even if you do eat something "unhealthy" your body will have time later to burn it off and then get back to burning stored fat. You'll never have to worry about going to dinner with friends and having to order a salad because you can eat what you want, as long as it's in your time frame.

"Suck it up now and you won't have to suck it in later!"

Health Benefits of The 16 Hour Diet

Now you know all of the great things that change in your body to help you burn fat fast, all by following The 16 Hour Diet. Sounds great, right? If this was the end of the story and The 16 Hour Diet didn't give any other benefits that would probably be enough for most people. But those aren't the only benefits from the diet. In fact, by not eating for an extended period of time, you actually gain a wide range of health benefits on top of losing weight. Sure, losing weight is probably your main goal, as it is mine. But after losing weight, it's important that your body is healthy so you can go out and enjoy life and your new body you've worked so hard for. Let's review just a few of the many health benefits you'll gain by following The 16 Hour Diet.

Detoxification and Cell Regeneration

When I say Detox, I don't mean anything like those products you see on TV or in the stores that claim to flush bad toxins from your body, but really just taste awful and do nothing. When I say detox, I mean the safe and natural process that your body actually performs on a daily basis. 24 hours a day your body is processing many different things that impact cells in your body, mainly cells called mitochondria. After cells have completed their life cycle, the body has a process called Autophagy to remove the worn out cells and replace them with new cells. This keeps the cells in your body fresh and full of life to continue to support your daily bodily functions. Remember, this is an important task that is constantly occurring in your body to keep up with the volume of cells you need to replace.

Now, this process occurs automatically and it happens 24 hours a day, but that doesn't mean it's working properly or even adequately enough to keep you healthy. A poor diet and being overweight can severely hinder the body's ability to replace worn out cells. Even if you are healthy, but you are constantly eating six small meals a day, your body is busy digesting your food and breaking it down to a cellular level, so it doesn't have time to take care of its other job of replacing old cells. Over time, your body creates a buildup of old worn out cells, which can make you feel and perform poorly and even lead to health problems. There are recent studies linking the lack of autophagy to diseases such as Huntington's and Alzheimer's, and poor cell regeneration is also linked to early aging.

With The 16 Hour Diet, you are giving your body time without digesting food, to focus solely on replacing outdated cells using autophagy. In addition, when you are in a fasted state, meaning you've gone longer than 12 hours without eating, then the autophagy process actually increase and becomes more efficient. There are also recent studies showing the connection between increased autophagy and fasting. This means that by following The 16 Hour Diet, your body becomes more efficient at the fundamental processes that keep us healthy and may even help prevent diseases related to aging.

Weight Loss

We've covered this already, but it bears repeating. The food you eat contains sugars to use as energy for your body. These sugars are stored in the liver as glycogen. Once your body stored the maximum amount of glycogen from your food, it begins storing any extra as fat. When the body needs energy, it first uses the full load of glycogen stores as energy, and if you're constantly eating, or even if you eat the basic 3 meals a day, your glycogen stores are constantly being refilled. It generally takes between 8-12 hours of no eating, for your body to completely deplete your glycogen stores and start burning stored fat cells for energy. This is why The 16 Hour Diet goes 16 hours without eating so you are guaranteed to deplete your glycogen stores and burn some serious fat cells. What does all this mean? It means you need to get ready to shop for a new wardrobe this summer!

Hormone Regulation

We've covered how certain hormones like HGH and specific enzymes that help to utilize those hormones to burn fat increase in production when you fast for longer than 12 hours. It's also important to note that HGH improves endurance while exercising, improves the time it takes to repair muscles, and increases the overall growth of muscles from working out. Did I mention that HGH also slows the aging process similar to the autophagy process also discussed earlier? One study showed that interval training while fasting increased HGH by 1300% in women and 2000% in men. Sounds great, right? All this comes from using The 16 Hour diet. Let's move on to some other hormones that are just as beneficial for losing weight and feeling great.

Leptin is a hormone that regulates fat storage as well as hunger signals. It's actually produced by fat cells and its purpose is to tell your brain to tell you to stop eating by shutting down your feeling of hunger. This happens once your body has reached a sufficient level of fat for survival and reproduction so that it may continue to live and thrive. Fat, as evil as you consider it, is actually necessary for survival, and you will always have a certain percent of your body made up of fat. This hormone is designed to keep you from losing all your fat by telling you to consume more for survival. Pretty cool how much actually happens in our body that we aren't really aware of. By the way, the reason that many low-fat diets fail is because they conflict with the natural physiology of our bodies and our own survival instinct. By restricting your body from fat, your body will only scream louder that you need it to survive, until you succumb and eat some.

So how does this tie into our 16 Hour diet? If fat is so good for survival, then why should I lose it? Well fat is needed to survive, but only a small percentage of your body, at most 7% is actually needed to thrive long term. 7% is ridiculously low for someone to maintain, and people with this amount of body fat will look absolutely ripped and toned, as if they don't have a shred of fat on them. However, many people, especially people who are overweight, can have up to 40% body fat. This level is extremely unhealthy and can and most likely will cause serious health problems and ultimately, death. Remember I said that fat cells actually produce Leptin to tell you you're full? So why do overweight just get this feeling and stop eating? Well, the issue is that your body is most likely screaming to you that its full, but your brain has become insensitive or tolerant to this signal due to the extensive amount of hormone Leptin that sits in your body at all times from the high fat level. In other words, you have so much Leptin in your body that you've become deaf to its signal and don't get that "full" feeling when you should.

The 16 Hour Diet is the perfect prescription to this issue. When you go longer than 12 hours without eating, you allow your body to completely digest all sugars and glycogen stores kept on hand. From that point, your body starts to balance out and start using fat cells as energy, as well as refreshing your cells via autophagy. The same triggers that cause fasting to kick start these processes, is the same that clears your brain in a way to start tuning back in to the Leptin signal. Over time, you reboot your body to hear the signals from Leptin that you should normally feel. Once you "reboot" your body, your Leptin signals will be heard loud and clear. This means that when you consume fat, after a certain point, you will feel full. This means that your cravings and constant feeling of hunger will disappear because your body will finally realize it has enough and doesn't need anymore. Once your cravings and hunger pangs are gone, you will feel free from food, and you'll only have to eat when you need to. At this point, you gain control of your diet and your body. When I reached this point, I felt truly empowered and its one of the main reasons I will continue The 16 Hour Diet forever.

Insulin Sensitivity

One of the biggest health benefits to The 16 Hour Diet is Insulin Sensitivity. Insulin is another hormone and its purpose is to signal your body to absorb blood glucose into muscles and tissues, where it is stored as glycogen for energy. When we eat, our insulin levels go up, and blood glucose enters our blood stream. By being insulin sensitive, our tissues are more receptive to absorbing the blood glucose, which means it is not lingering in our blood stream, and instead is being used by our muscles for activity. The problem comes when you are constantly eating foods and providing sugar into your body. The first thing that happens is that you are constantly producing insulin. Like we saw with Leptin, the longer your body constantly produces a hormone, the more likely you are to build a tolerance to it, meaning its purpose or use is less effective or nonexistent completely. Over time, your body stops responding to the insulin, so then your muscles don't absorb the blood glucose for energy. This is also known as Insulin Resistance. If your muscles are absorbing it, then it can only go one place, and that is to stay in your blood stream. This is a very bad place to keep sugars for an extended period of time. High levels of blood glucose have been linked to nearly every chronic disease and are a main cause of diseases such as Diabetes and other heart disease.

Now I know for a fact that no one wants diabetes, so let's talk about how The 16 Hour Diet can help prevent it. When you go 16 hours without eating, your body stops consuming sugars from food, which means eventually your body stops producing insulin. This allows your body to reset from its recent insulin intake and await the next round of insulin from the next time you eat. After a few times of this start and stop process, your body starts to become increasingly sensitive to the insulin. This is because you go more time without insulin so your body starts to look for it more aggressively. When insulin finally does come in, your body quickly consumes and converts it for the proper processes. This is more commonly referred to as Insulin Sensitivity, which is much better than the resistance and tolerance, and is a goal among many diets tailored specifically for diabetes. Another benefit to being insulin sensitive is that, when your insulin levels shut off, your pancreas reacts by stopping its production and conversion of blood glucose. This is good because, if you remember, it's the blood glucose sitting in the blood stream that causes diabetes. Therefore, if we limit and reduce the amount our body produces, we reduce our overall risk of diabetes.

So to recap, using The 16 Hour Diet causes our body to become insulin sensitive which improves the overall benefits of insulin, and reduces the amount of blood glucose we produce that would otherwise sit in our blood stream and cause disease. This process of reducing the stagnant glucose in our blood stream is the reason why this diet helps reduce our risk of diabetes and other chronic diseases and in some cases can reverse diabetes and high blood pressure.

"You can push harder every day because you're worth it. Every single effort you make is changing your body and making you healthier inside and out. Never give up!"

Turbo Charge

Now we've covered the main aspects of The 16 Hour Diet. With this information, you will safely and effectively lose weight and will reach your goals finally! That is reason for celebration! I have however, kept a few tricks up my sleeve that can ramp up your weight loss efforts and Turbo Charge your overall results. This section is dedicated specifically to boosting The 16 Hour Diet and is designed for those who are willing to do every single thing they can to lose weight and meet their goals faster. You can use one or all of the tips listed below. It's based on your comfort level and how quickly you want to lose weight. I would suggest starting the basic plan of The 16 Hour Diet first, before stepping into this section. Once you can comfortably fast for at least 16 Hours, you can graduate and begin implanting these incredible tools for Turbo Charging your weight loss. Let's get started with my favorite way to boost results.

Increase the amount of hours you fast

One sure fire way to turbo charge your weight loss results is to extend the amount of time you go without eating. The 16 Hour Diet asks that you go at least 16 hours each day without eating. Once you're comfortable and can achieve this without issue, why not try kicking that to 17 or 18 hours. If you're feeling brave, go 20 hours without eating, and then eat for 4 hours and then fast for another 20. You can even do this once or twice a week, and work your way up to every day if you'd like. This can be done safely as long as you still eat enough calories within those 4 hours. Refer back to the calorie calculator and your weight loss goals to determine how much you need to eat during those 4 hours. I covered earlier in the book the benefits of fasting and how your body starts using your stored fat for energy. So it makes sense that the longer you fast, the more time your body has to use up stored fat for energy. I usually fast for 20 hours at least one day every week, and my husband does this consistently during the summer months to burn extra fat. Just remember to eat enough during your shortened window of eating. It may be tough for some people to eat 1500 calories in 4 hours.

Exercise before you eat your first meal of the day

This is my favorite way to turbo charge weight loss results and is a great way to get in shape and build muscle. Do your daily exercise routine after you have fasted for at least 12 hours but before you eat your first meal of the day. Exercising while in a fasted state increases the amount of fat you burn during activity because your body has no food stores to convert to the energy needed. Even better is that after you complete your workout routine, your body will stay in this supercharged fat burning mode for an additional couple of hours. Don't worry about needing food to fuel your workouts, or needing some type of pre-workout drink or meal bar. Claims about needing to eat before exercise are unfounded and there is no clinical support for them. The truth is your body has plenty of fuel already stored in the fat cells you carry. This is the physiological purpose of fat cells, to be able to provide us with energy if there is no food in our bodies to burn through. Therefore, you should feel free and easy about working out as hard as you like without eating any food beforehand. I highly recommend incorporating weight training and high intensity interval training into your workout routine. The more muscle you build on your body, the more calories you will burn throughout the day and you'll also look more toned overall.

Along with burning additional fat, exercising while fasted also utilizes some of the benefits of fasting. For example, we've discussed that fasting increases the body's production of HGH naturally. HGH is basically like steroids, but it's a safe and natural hormone our bodies produce, and one of its purposes is to help the body build quality muscle. If you're already producing more HGH by fasting, you might as well put it to good use by lifting weights and working out. Everybody wants a sexy toned body to strut at the beach, and this is one sure fire way to get it. When you're done working out and finally decide to eat your first meal, the fact that you exercised while fasted continues to give benefits. Doing this actually improves the body's effectiveness in synthesizing nutrients from the food you eat. Basically, working out while fasted helps your body become more efficient at processing the food, once you decide to eat. This means that the vitamins and nutrients that are normally in your food will be absorbed better into your body and blood stream, and provide a better benefit to you long term. This is a very key fact when it comes to protein. Protein is a key macronutrient that your body needs to survive and thrive and is also the key main component to building muscle. Working out while fasted improves protein synthesis and absorption into the muscle fibers, so you get the full impact of it.

All in all, exercising and more specifically weight training while fasted, brings many additional benefits to help you turbo charge your weight loss. I love that my body is finally working for me and not against me. I personally couldn't believe the results I was getting from this tip. Yes, working out is hard when your overweight and out of shape, and it can be a nightmare to some people. This is a magical tip because the quicker we start losing our fat, the easier it will become for us to move around and workout!

Drink more water

This is the easiest way to boost weight loss and is also important to your overall health. It's also the one that most of us forget to do. All you have to do is to drink more water. How much, you ask? Well a good rule to follow is to drink half your weight in ounces of water daily. So if you weigh 160 pounds, then you should drink 80 ounces of water on a daily basis. Why does this turbo charge weight loss? Well this helps for a few reasons. One is that hydrating your body with water is crucial for many different pasts of your body. Americans in general are dehydrated because they don't drink enough water. This can cause your body to become bloated and can affect the ratio of nutrients in your bloodstream. Also, drinking water can suppress appetite, and even replace it in some cases. The feeling of thirst can be easily mistaken as hunger in the brain. If you don't like drinking water, try adding some zero calorie sweeteners to your water. These sweeteners can dramatically change the flavor of your water so that it tastes more like juice, but you still get the same hydrating benefit. There are so many products in stores now that work for this. So next time you feel hungry during your fast, do a quick water check and see if you've drank enough water that day. You could just be thirsty. Also drinking ice water increases the amount of calories your body burns. That's right drinking ice cold water helps burn calories! I love that.

Eat clean foods

So this one is pretty basic, but it needs to be covered. We've already said that you don't need to count calories and you cans still enjoy the foods you love while doing The 16

Hour Diet. However, we've also said that the basic formula for weight loss is the calories you consume – calories you burn through exercise and the daily calories your body burns. So then it makes perfect sense that if you're eating foods that are high in calories and fats, that you will either need to eat extremely less food, or you'll end up consuming too many calories and not losing weight. Even worse, you may end up gaining weight. Foods that are fried or covered in creamy sauces can be guaranteed to be loaded with calories. Basically any meal on a restaurant menu will have more calories than you probably think. Unless the restaurant provides the calories on the menu, you can probably assume that meal you're about to order is at least 1000 calories, but is probably even higher than that. There are so many websites now that provide calorie info for basically every meal you can order at a restaurant. Next time you go out to eat, go ahead and order your favorite meal, but check online to see how many calories it has. You may be surprised at what you see.

So what should you do then, if so many delicious foods are loaded with calories? Well, something I've already recommended as an easy first step is to drop sugary soda and switch to diet. Not only can you drink diet soda while you're fasting, but by eliminating caloric drinks, you can save those calories for foods that can actually provide nutrients to your body. I never drink my calories unless I'm having a treat like a smoothie, or maybe a margarita ;). Next thing you can do is to stay away from fried foods. Instead, order your chicken grilled or blackened, and order your veggie and sides steamed. Doing this alone can dramatically reduce the amount of calories in your meal. Some days I even trade my waffle fries for a side salad. Remember it's the small steps and changing little things that will eventually add up to big changes in your habits and in the way your body looks on the outside.

Now let me clarify that when I say clean, I'm not referring to eating brown rice with a small piece of plain tilapia, and a few pieces of boiled broccoli. That is a clean meal, but you'll eventually go crazy from the lack of flavor and excitement. Also, eating like that on a regular basis, at least for me, is not sustainable. That's the reason those super restrictive diets are so hard to stick to and we eventually give up on them. When I say clean, I mean eating some homemade black bean soup, or chicken stir-fry. I list some great and clean recipes at the end of the book. Try some of these and I'm sure you'll enjoy eating clean foods and you'll also enjoy the slimmer waist line as well.

Use safe and natural supplements

Let me start by saying many of the weight loss "supplements" you will find in stores do not work, and should not even be considered supplements. They're more like placebo's, or even better, a complete waste of money. This also goes for diet pills, so stay away from anything that's getting front row in your local supermarket. The supplements I provide below are natural and found in nature and assist the body in its normal processes that burn fat, most of which we've covered already. These can be taken safely and without worry of dangerous side effects, and will certainly help you turbo charge your weight loss. When looking to purchase these supplements, be sure to go to your local supermarkets and vitamin shops. Avoid the internet or anyone trying to sell you them with claims that you will become slimmer overnight. A lot of the items online will advertise to have the key supplement I mention below but they may really only contain trace amounts of what you want, and may actually contain unhealthy chemical additives. I can find all of these at my local stores and they're affordable and come in the doses I recommend below.

CLA

CLA stands for conjugated linoleic acid and is a fatty acid found in some meats. Yes, this is a fat that is good for you, and good fats do exist. CLA helps the body by facilitating the process of opening and releasing fat from your fat cells. The easier it is to release fat, the easier and more effectively your body will burn that fat way. CLA can be found in the vitamin section of your local grocery store or Wal-Mart, and is very inexpensive. I recommend taking at least 3,000mg's every day an hour before you work out. Doing this before a workout is just another way to help increase the amount of fat you burn.

Forskolin

Forskolin is another natural supplement found in nature, and can be found in the roots of an herb in the mint family. Clinical studies have shown that Forskolin can help break down fat cells, meaning releasing and burning fat. It can also help remove fat from adipose tissue, which is harder fat cells to reach, and will also help build lean muscle. This supplement can be more difficult to find, so check with your local vitamin shops and health food stores. Make sure you find a bottle with 20% Forskolin, which is the "good stuff" and try to take 125 mg's per day of the Forskolin. I have great results from all of these supplements but I believe this one really helps the scale go down.

Garcinia Cambogia

Garcinia is the hottest new supplement going around town. It's a fruit found in Southeast Asia and helps to burn fat and build muscle. I can attest that this supplement helps burn fat. This fruit, and more importantly the extract, has new clinical studies to support its effects on weight loss, and can help increase your body's weight loss ability by two to three times. No diet pill currently on market can make that claim and back it up with science. This supplement does a few things for your body. First, it increases serotonin, which helps with your mood and emotions and overall makes you feel happier. It also helps manage cortisol, which helps you manage stress. If you didn't already know, stress, anxiety, and lack of sleep are three contributors to weight gain, and three challenges to overcome when trying to lose weight. Stress alone is also a major contributor to belly fat, which is many peoples biggest problem area.

Those are great benefits alone, but this supplement does more. Garcinia helps by communicating to your liver to take the foods you've eaten and help convert them to glycogen to be used immediately as energy, instead of creating fat to store in your fat cells. Basically, it helps block the body from creating and storing fat. On top of that, it helps decrease your appetite so you consume less fat and calories overall. Last but not least, it helps create lean muscle mass which helps increase the amount of calories your body burns naturally. Combine all these items, and you're left with a fat burning miracle supplement that is safe and natural, and will surely help you turbo charge your weight loss and meet your goals. This can be found in your local vitamin shops. You should look for Garcinia, also referred to as GCE (Garcinia Cambogia Extract) that has 50% HCA, which is the actual extract from the rind of the fruit. Also, be sure it comes with Potassium, which will help the extract be absorbed into the bloodstream more effectively. You should take at least 3,000mg's day and take it about one hour before you eat your first meal of the day. I take it when I wake up in the mornings this way I insure it has time to take effect on my body and its a few hours before I eat.

These three supplements, CLA, Forskolin, and Garcinia, have worked miracles on me and I still take them every day. If you use these in conjunction with The 16 Hour Diet, you'll be amazed by the way you look! I know you're ready to look your best, and I'm so excited to share these secrets with you. ☺

"Start where you are. Use what you have. Do what you can."

Ready, Set, Go!

So, there it is! Now you know all about The 16 Hour Diet and how it helps you lose weight and turn your body in to a FAT burning machine. You know how fasting changes your body and the great health benefits it provides. You also know more about losing weight and how you can finally reach your weight loss goals. You also now have some great supplements that can help you along the way and turbo charge your weight loss. So, what next? Where do you go from here? This section is all about summarizing what we've learned and exactly what you need to do to start your weight loss journey. After reading this section, you will be able to begin immediately and start feeling great and have the body and live the life you've always wanted.

"I am not telling you it's going to be easy, I am telling you it's going to be worth it!"

Expectations

Before I let you loose on the world and on your journey to your ideal body, let's first talk about what you should expect when following The 16 Hour Diet. Expectations are great, but high expectations have killed some of the greatest thought, ideas, and plans people have had. I've been on diet fads before that promise you will lose 10 pounds in the first week. Well, guess what; I didn't lose 10 pounds, or even one pound, and I was completely bummed out about it. Needless to say, I didn't give that diet a second look afterward. On the flip side, if I told you that this rigid diet will require you to completely change your life so you can eat this specific way, but you should only expect to lose two pounds, no one wants to hear that either. No one has the time or patience to put that much work into a diet, only to expect such little weight loss. With The 16 Hour Diet, I want you to understand and expect that you don't have to give up eating the foods you love, but you can still expect to lose a healthy amount of weight at a rate that will excite and motivate you to keep going.

That is what makes The 16 Hour Diet so great. So far, I haven't guaranteed you will lose 20 pounds the first month, and I won't say that, because it's not realistic, or healthy for that matter. Also every person is different and will lose weight differently. Therefore, it's unreasonable to set that expectation. However, the good news is that there's also no low floor, like 1 pound a month. The 16

Hour Diet is great in that, with the basic plan, and the Turbo Charge ideas, you can control how much you lose by basing it on how much you want to put into the plan. If you only want to fast for 16 hours a day, and stick to your normal diet and caloric intake, then you will lose a certain amount. If you decide to take it to the max and fast for 17-20 hours a day, take natural supplements, work out while you're fasted, and eat healthy, clean foods, then you can expect to lose more. I lost 12 pounds my first month of fasting.

With The 16 Hour Diet, and fasting in general, it normally takes at least 2 weeks, but can take some people up to 4 weeks to start seeing results. That is because the health benefits and physiology we've discussed doesn't just change overnight. Your body and brain are way smarter than that, and no better than to change everything after one day of difference. It takes these 2-4 weeks for your body to adjust to this change in routine and start doing the things we've discussed, such as utilizing fat stores for energy. Think about, this whole time you've been alive, your body has grown used to you eating every few hours so it depends on this and nothing else for the energy you need. Your body won't change unless it's thoroughly convinced that it needs to. Once your body learns that you will be going 16 Hours without eating, it will appropriately adjust to start utilizing fat stores for energy. Some people get discouraged after the first few weeks when they don't lose any weight, so this is an important fact to know. Remember, this is not a fad diet, but a way of living that allows you to lose weight, be healthy, and enjoy life by continuing to eat the foods you love.

The normal guideline for healthy weight loss that's sustainable is to lose one to two pounds per week. A good rule of thumb that I follow is to divide your current weight by 100 and make that your weekly goal in pounds for losing weight. If you weigh 200 pounds now, then your weekly goal would be 2 pounds per week. Now remember, this is your goal expectation. That means that if you don't hit that goal one week, that is your indicator you can probably be doing more to meet the goal. Maybe you didn't fast for 16 hours straight for a few days that week. Or maybe you've reached a point where fasting alone may not be enough, so you should consider exercise, or one of the Turbo Charge ideas. Either way, following The 16 Hour Diet means that you can expect to lose weight every week, and no matter how much it turns out to be, losing some is better than losing none. The 16 Hour Diet is meant to be a sustainable and enjoyable way of living that allows you to eat the foods you love, have time to enjoy life, and be able to live healthy with the body you deserve to have without stressing and going bananas.

"A goal without a plan is a wish!"

S.M.A.R.T. Goal

The SMART Goal has been around forever and is a tried and true management principle that has been helping people succeed for years. SMART is an acronym that stands for Specific, Measurable, Attitude, Realistic and Time-specific. I want you to use the SMART technique when you set your weight loss goals and expectation. Not only that, but go ahead and use it in your everyday life as a way to get ahead and be successful. Here are some ways to set SMART goals for each of the categories.

Specific – Specific means that your goal is clearly defined with no grey area. That means that, instead of saying you're going to lose weight every week, say that you're going to lose exactly two pounds every week. This way, if you don't hit the two pound mark, then you can go back and reassess why and make adjustments, so that next week you will hit that goal. A great way to ensure your goal is specific is to ask the 'W' questions:

- What: What do I want to accomplish?
    - Obviously, this one will be losing weight, but please be sure to make the goal and number specific, both for your overall ideal weight, and the amount of weight you want to lose each week.
- Why: Specific reasons, purpose, or benefits of accomplishing the goal.
    - We talked about setting your Why's and now they come into play here. Be sure you have your whys as they will keep you accountable and motivated.
- Who: Who will be involved?
    - Of course you're going to be involved, but maybe you want your best friend to come along

and share your journey. Or maybe, you want your husband and family to follow The 16 Hour Diet in order to keep eating times set to fit your plan. Specify these things here.
- Where: Identify a location.
    - Will you work out at home, or get a gym membership? Will you only eat at home, or will you go out to eat when you're not fasting?
- Which: Identify requirements and challenges
    - This is where you list the things in your life that need to change or that may get in the way of your 16 Hour diet. Does your lunch time at work come when you will be fasting? This is a great example of a challenge a lot of people face, so try to find a

way to work around this, or just fast until work ends☺.

Measurable – Your goal needs to be measurable to ensure you can track and confirm if you're meeting the goal. The good news for us is that losing weight is very measureable. All you have to do is jump on the scale to see if the pounds came off. But, maybe you want to add waist inches to your goal, as well as pounds. For most people they do see inches coming off when the scale is not moving. Or maybe you want to measure how many days you fast for 16 hours, and how many days you fast for less or more. All of these are great things to track, and the more information you track, the better informed you become about your weight loss needs.

Attitude – This is my favorite of the SMART categories. Attitude is all about how you view your weight loss journey, how you view The 16 Hour Diet, and how you view yourself. If you have a bad outlook on any of these things, chances are you won't be as successful as you could be. However, if you are excited about losing weight, and excited about living healthy and having the body of your dreams, then your weight loss will reflect this. Remember, stress can affect your weight loss, or worse, cause you to gain weight. Having a great attitude will carry you past your challenges and help you manage stress along your journey. Stress, anger, and disappointment are only a mindset, and are a choice. You can choose to feel this way, or you can choose to feel awesome and excited about what you're doing.

Realistic – This is really here as a reality check to see if what you've set for your SMART goal so far, is actually going to work. Simply ask yourself; is this goal realistic? If your goal is to lose 10 pounds a week, and you're only going to fast for 14 hours day with no exercise or diet change, that goal is not realistic. If you are 5'10" tall and your "ideal weight" is 110 pounds, that also is not realistic. Make sure that your goals and expectations are realistic given yourself and your environment. More importantly, remember that being realistic does not mean you can't be ambitious!

Time-specific – This one is crucial when you're losing weight. It's great to say that you will lose 2 pounds week, and you want to weigh 160 pounds as your ideal weight. But if you don't set a date to your target weight, then if you come across challenges, or fall behind, there is no barrier at the end that will keep you accountable and motivated. Another reason to set a time for your weight loss is that you can tell others in your support group, so they too can keep you accountable. Even better, giving an end date for your goal can help give you the deserved closure to your amazing weight loss journey, so you can look back and celebrate the hard work you've done, and the amazing results you've had.

Here is a sample SMART goal below. Use this as an example when setting your goal to make sure you've covered everything.

"I want to lose 40 pounds in 6 months. I want to do this by losing 2 pounds per week. The reason I want to do this is because I want to feel great in my bathing suit during our summer vacation to the beach. My husband will also do The 16 Hour Diet with me so we can eat during the same times, and I'll be working out at home. I have a newborn baby, so I'll need to find time to work out between nap times, or when my husband gets home. I'm going to weigh in every Monday morning to check my progress, and assess the past week with my food journal where I will keep track of everything I eat. My goal is very realistic and I'm super excited to look great when we go to the beach."

"A huge part of losing weight is believing you can do it and realizing it's not going to happen overnight."

Recap

Now that you have your expectations and SMART goals set, you're almost ready to get started. Let's recap the main points of what we've learned and what you need to do to lose weight with The 16 Hour Diet.

- Set your "Why" to keep you on track and motivated during tough times
- A 'Fasted' state is reached when you go 12 straight hours without eating. The 16 Hour Diet asks you not to eat for at least 16 straight hours to see optimal weight loss results.
- Fasting works because you give your body time to burn through its food

stores (glycogen) and then start using stored fat as energy, turning your body into a Fat Burning machine!
- Fasting also provides many other health benefits such as insulin sensitivity, hormone regulation, and autophagy
- The 16 Hour Diet allows you to lose weight while still enjoying the foods you love, because it focuses on making your body work for you and burn more fat than it normally would
- Turbo Charge your weight loss by fasting longer than 16 hours, working out while fasted, taking supplements, and eating clean and healthy
- Set your SMART goals and expectations to ensure you're successful in losing weight

"Wake up with Determination. Go to bed with satisfaction."

First 3 steps to get started

We've come to the end, and it's almost time to let you free on your weight loss journey. You're ready to turn your body into a fat burning machine and make it work for you to lose pounds easily and effectively. To make sure you get off to an amazing start, here are 3 simple steps to get you started and on the road to the body of your dreams.

1. Set your Why
    - I've said it a bunch, but it's the most important key to success. Set your Why and keep it handy so you can constantly be reminded of why you're on this incredible journey

2. Set your SMART goal and calculate your 'Caloric Maintenance' number
    - Manage expectations and keep yourself accountable with a SMART goals. Use my formula to calculate your caloric needs so you know how much you should be eating to lose weight.
3. Pick your time of day to start The 16 Hour Diet
    - Decide what day you're going to start and pick the time of day to have dinner and stop eating. Then from that time, don't eat for at least 12 hours, and try working your way up each day until you can go 16 straight hours without eating. When it's time to eat again, eat like you normally would for 8 hours, and then start you're The 16 Hour Diet again.

These 3 steps are all you need to get started with The 16 Hour Diet. Thank you so much for buying and reading my book. I truly hope that it helps you lose weight and have the body and life you deserve, just like it helped me. Keep reading below for great recipe ideas for eating healthy, as well as an FAQ section for common questions. Thanks again and congratulations on losing weight!

"It takes 4 weeks for you to see your body changing. It takes 8 weeks for your family and friends. It takes 12 weeks for the rest of the world. KEEP GOING!"

Frequently Asked Questions

Q: When do my 16 hours actually begin?

A: Here's the simplest way to think about it: Your 16 Hour Diet starts after you finish eating your last meal of the day. If you finish dinner by 6pm, then your 16 hours starts at 6pm and goes until 10am the next morning, when you can eat your first meal of the day.

Q: Do I have to use the same exact times every day for this diet to work?

A: No, you can move your hours as you like or need. Maybe one day you fast for 16 Hours, and the next you fast for 20 hours, and then go to 18 hours the third day. Each of these days, you will be eating and stopping at different times, and that's okay. The point is for the majority of the week, you go at least 16 hours straight without eating a single calorie.

Q: What if I can't go 16 Hours one day, or what if I want to take a day off one day?

A: This diet is great because it's flexible. If you want to cut down from 16 Hours to 12 hours, or even take a day off, then go ahead and do it. A cheat day can help keep you focused and on track, helping you stick to the diet for the long run. I usually have a cheat day once every two weeks where I don't fast at all, and I eat any and all foods I want to eat. Just make sure it doesn't turn into a weekly or daily habit. Remember that every decision you make will impact your goals and dreams one way or another, so be conscious about making the best decisions every day.

Q: Can I eat anything during my 16 Hour Diet?

A: No, during the 16 Hours of fasting, the main objective is to deplete your food stores so your body can start using your stored fat as energy. In order to begin this process, you must go at least 12 hours, but we recommend 16 hours, without eating any food. This includes healthy foods such as veggies.

Q: Not even a celery stick?

A: No, not even a celery stick.

Q: I've been following the diet but I haven't lost any weight. What should I do?

A: Has it been longer than 4 weeks? Remember that for some people, it can take up to 4 weeks for our bodies to acknowledge this change of not eating and then begin the process of breaking down fat cells for energy in an efficient manner. If it's been longer than 4 weeks, stop and assess what you've been doing and then compare to what I recommend in the book. Are you burning more calories throughout the day than you are consuming? Are you tracking and measuring your decisions and progress on a daily and weekly basis? Are you fasting for at least 16 hours consistently? If yes to these questions, you should consider one or all of the Turbo Charge suggestions. It could be that you're at a point where your body needs the additional push to continue losing weight.

Q: What can I do to curb hunger pains when I'm fasting?

A: Here are some great ways to curb hunger when you first start fasting. Remember that eventually those hunger pains will subside, because fasting actually helps suppress appetite. While your body adjusts, you can drink zero calorie drinks such as diet soda because caffeine can suppress appetite. You can also drink water, lots of water, and try adding some zero calorie sweetener. Try chewing sugar-free gum if you feel the need to chew or "eat" something. Lastly, if you just can't shake the hunger, try exercising or focus on your daily tasks. Keeping your body busy and providing healthy stimulation can help suppress appetite.

Q: What if I like to drink alcohol when I go out on weekends at night?

A: Same policy, only zero calorie drinks are allowed during your 16 Hour fast. Try drinking a Vodka and diet soda, which is zero calories and quite tasty!

Q: I work nights, so I can't start my diet at the suggested times. What should I do?

A: The great thing about The 16 Hour Diet is that you can choose and adjust the times as needed. Just make sure the majority of your 16 hour diet occurs while you're sleeping. This way, you can fast while you're sleeping, and eat while you're active in your day and burning calories.

Q: I thought breakfast was the "most important meal of the day" because it kick-starts your metabolism. If breakfast is so important for me, why should I skip it?

A: Let me start by saying there is no actual scientific research or clinical studies that prove that breakfast helps boost metabolism in any way. The truth is that your metabolism is pretty constant and isn't necessarily influenced by eating meals. This also is true for the "eat 6 small meals a day" trend in dieting. There is no science to back that claim as actually improving metabolism either. The only scientifically proven way to actually increase your metabolic rate is to increase lean muscle mass on your body. This is because muscle burns more calories that fat, so increasing the amount of muscle you have will increase the amount of calories your body burns.

Q: What about breakfast giving me energy to start my day?

Again, another myth about breakfast that isn't entirely rooted in truth. The truth is that our body determines how much energy it actually needs when it needs it. If there is no food in our body to use as fuel, our body starts to convert stored fat into energy. This is the physiological reason why our bodies store fat to begin with. The 16 Hour Diet helps you lose weight because it gives your body time to go through this natural process, instead of constantly filling yourself with food.

Q: When it's time for me to eat, should I still try to have 3 square meals, or 6 small meals during my 8 hours?

A: No, it doesn't matter how many meals you have. What matters is how many calories you consume during your 8 hours. If you don't consume enough calories, or if you consume too many calories, you will hamper your weight loss. Remember the formula for losing weight; Weight loss = Calories you consume – Calories you burn. Nowhere in that formula does it specify how many meals to eat. ☺

Q: Can I use Stevia or Sweet-N -Low for my coffee/tea during my 16 Hour Diet?

A: Yes, you can use any zero calorie sweeteners for any zero calorie drinks.

Q: Where can I go if I have additional questions?

A: Connect with us on social media for more great info, answers and encouragement on your weight loss journey.

"Never give up! Everyone has bad days. Pick yourself up and KEEP GOING!"

<u>Bonus Recipes</u>

Here are my easy recipes for turbo charged weight loss. These are all packed with foods to help your body work for you. I love each and every one, and yes, these are my personal meals that I use at home. I've used these meals to help me lose weight and I still use these in conjunction with The 16 Hour Diet! When it comes to eating, I think you should remember that you need to enjoy your food, so make small healthier choices each time you eat, and eventually eating healthy will be what you want to do. As you start this diet, remember to make your meals easy. Don't stress over every detail. You can use frozen veggies and still be healthy. The key is to make it easy make it fun and enjoy every meal. Lastly, this is not a diet you need to follow with The 16 Hour Diet. These are simply suggestions in case you're looking for new and healthy meal ideas. As I said earlier, you don't need to drastically change the way you eat in order to lose weight, but if you want lose weight fast, eating clean and healthy will definitely help.

Chocolate-Dipped Banana Bites

Chocolate is a rich source of Yummy! Bananas are the richest source of resistant starch, a type of healthy carbohydrate that helps you burn calories and eat less. Yummy + Healthy makes this dessert snack a weight-loss winner.

Ingredients:
2 tablespoons semisweet chocolate chips/ or dark chocolate
1 small banana, peeled and cut into 1-inch chunks

Preparation"
1. Place chocolate chips in a small microwave-safe bowl. Microwave at HIGH 1 minute or until chocolate melts. Dip banana pieces in chocolate.

Upbeat egg salad sandwich

The curry in this Upbeat egg salad adds a health-promoting antioxidant jolt to this traditional southern comfort dish. The Low fat yogurt saves on calories verses traditional mayonnaise that most people like myself put in egg salad.

Ingredients:
2 hard-cooked eggs, chopped
2 tablespoons plain Greek-style low-fat yogurt
2 tablespoons chopped red bell pepper
2 tablespoons chopped onion
1/4 teaspoon curry powder
1/8 teaspoon salt
1/8 teaspoon pepper
2 slices of your favorite bread, toasted
1/2 cup fresh spinach

Preparation:

1. Combine eggs, yogurt, bell pepper, onion, curry powder, salt, and pepper, in a small bowl; Mix well.

2. Place spinach on your favorite bread, top with egg salad, and enjoy this southern comfort sandwich.

Spicy Southern Black Bean Soup.

Black beans are packed with protein. Cilantro contains high levels of antioxidants and acts as a digestive aid and it fights cellulite making this Spicy Southern Black Bean Soup a Fat fighting dish!!

Ingredients:
1 large chopped onion (about 1 1/2 cups
1 cup jalapeno, seeded and chopped
1 large garlic clove, finely chopped
2 tablespoons chili powder
1 teaspoon ground cumin

 32 ounces can roasted red pepper and tomato soup (or tomato soup)
2 (15.5 ounce) cans black beans, rinsed and drained
1/4 cup reduced-fat sour cream
1/4 cup chopped fresh cilantro
 Add avocado and Cilantro (optional)

Preparation:

1. In a pre-heated pan add the onion and jalapeño cook, stirring until softened (about 3 minutes). Stir in the garlic, chili powder, and cumin cook 1 minute. Stir in soup and black beans simmer 5 minutes. Stir in the chopped cilantro.

2. Ladle soup into bowls top with 1 tablespoon of sour cream, avocado, and cilantro, if desired.

Southwestern Pizza

Ingredients:
Nonstick cooking spray
1 12-inch 100% whole wheat pizza crust
1 cup prepared tomato salsa
1 1/4 cups shredded reduced-fat 2 percent mozzarella
1 1/3 cups canned black beans, drained and rinsed
1 small sweet red pepper, seeded and thinly sliced (about 2/3 cup)
2 scallions, trimmed and thinly sliced
1/4 cup cilantro leaves for garnish (optional)

Preparation:
1. Heat the oven to 450 degrees. Coat a baking sheet with cooking spray. Place crust on sheet and top with salsa, 1 cup mozzarella, beans, sliced red pepper, and scallions. Top with remaining 1/4 cup cheese.
2. Place pizza in oven and bake 8 to 10 minutes or until mozzarella is melted. Remove from oven and garnish with cilantro if desired.

Easy Omelet night

Use either fresh or frozen broccoli. Both work just fine. The feta cheese adds some CLAs plus a punch of flavor, too. You can play with this and add the veggies you love changing it up every night if you like!

Ingredients:
Cooking spray
1 cup chopped broccoli
2 large eggs, beaten
2 tablespoons feta cheese, crumbled
1/4 teaspoon dried dill
2 slices bread, toasted

Preparation:
1. Heat a nonstick skillet over medium heat. Coat pan with cooking spray. Add broccoli, and cook 3 minutes.

2. Combine egg, feta, and dill in a small bowl. Add egg mixture to pan. Cook 3 to 4 minutes; flip omelet and cook 2 minutes or until cooked through. Serve with toast.

One pan Chicken Dinner

Ingredients:

4 boneless skinless chicken breast

2 pounds of green beans or you could use 2 cans of your favorite green beans

1 small onion

1 small bag of red skin potatoes

1 pack of Zesty Italian dressing mix

Preparation:
1. In your Pan 9x13 place your green beans with chopped onion on the bottom of pan coat with olive oil, salt, and pepper. Then add your halved potatoes and then place the chicken on the top. Cover with foil and bake at 350 for 1 hour

Oatmeal chocolate peanut butter clumps
These tasty clusters offer up two appetite-suppressing ingredients: The oatmeal contains resistant starch, and the dark chocolate is full of healthy fats to help curb cravings. Peanut butter provides protein. What more could you ask for RIGHT?

Ingredients:
2 tablespoons peanut butter
2 tablespoons 1% low-fat milk
1/4 cup semisweet chocolate chips
3/4 cup old-fashioned rolled oats

Preparation:
1. Heat peanut butter, milk, and chocolate chips in a saucepan over low heat 3 minutes or until chips melt.

2. Stir in oats. Remove from heat.

3. With a spoon, drop 8 ball-shaped portions on a wax paper–lined baking sheet. Let set in fridge 10 minutes. Sooooo yummy you will love this snack.

Veggie Tacos

This low-cal taco adds a kick with the addition of jalapeño peppers adding spice increases the amount of calories your body burns during digestion. Plus the veggies and beans add filling fiber and protein.

Ingredients:
2 red bell peppers, chopped
1 medium onion, chopped
1 cup sliced fresh mushrooms
1 to 2 jalapeño peppers, seeded and chopped
2 garlic cloves, minced
2 teaspoons olive oil
1 1/2 teaspoons ground cumin
1 teaspoon dried oregano
3/4 cup sweet white wine
1 (15-ounce) can pinto beans, rinsed and drained
2 cups chopped fresh spinach.
12 (8-inch) fat-free flour tortillas, warmed

1/2 cup crumbled reduced-fat feta cheese (optional) So yummy!

Preparation:

1. Sauté first 5 ingredients in hot oil in a skillet over medium-high heat 5 minutes or until vegetables are tender. Add cumin and oregano; sauté 2 minutes.

2. Stir in wine; reduce heat, and simmer 10 minutes or until liquid is reduced by half. Add beans, and cook until thoroughly heated. Add spinach; cook 2 minutes or until spinach wilts. Serve in warm tortillas with cheese, if desired.

Chicken and Guacamole tostada

This is my favorite dish. Guacamole has great healthy fats and chicken is packed with muscle building protein, making this meal perfect for losing weight.

Ingredients:

1 ripe peeled avocado

1 cup plus 2 tablespoons finely chopped tomato

3 tablespoons minced fresh onion

3 tablespoons fresh lime juice

1/2 teaspoon salt

1 small garlic clove, minced

1 tablespoon chopped fresh cilantro

1 tablespoon minced seeded jalapeño pepper

2 cups shredded skinless, boneless rotisserie chicken breast

1/4 teaspoon smoked paprika

8 (6-inch) corn tostada shells

Preparation:

1. Place avocado in a small bowl; mash with a fork. Stir in 2 tablespoons tomato, 1 tablespoon onion, 1 tablespoon juice, 1/4 teaspoon salt, and garlic.

2. Combine remaining 1 cup tomato, 2 tablespoons onion, 1 tablespoon lime juice, 1/4 teaspoon salt, cilantro, and jalapeño; toss well.

3. Combine chicken, remaining 1 tablespoon juice, and paprika; toss well to combine. Spread about 1 tablespoon guacamole over each tostada shell; top each with 1/4 cup chicken mixture and about 2 tablespoons salsa.

Zesty Chicken Salad

Ingredients:
Dressing:

1/3 cup chopped fresh cilantro

2/3 cup light sour cream

1 tablespoon minced chipotle chile, canned in adobo sauce

1 teaspoon ground cumin

1 teaspoon chili powder

4 teaspoons fresh lime juice

1/4 teaspoon salt

Salad:

4 cups shredded romaine lettuce

1 cup spinach leaves

2 cups chopped roasted skinless, boneless chicken breasts (about 2 breasts)

1 cup cherry tomatoes, halved

Some diced avocado

1/3 cup thinly vertically sliced red onion

1 (15-ounce) can black beans, rinsed and drained

1 (8 3/4-ounce) can no-salt-added whole-kernel corn, rinsed and drained

Preparation:

1. To prepare dressing, combine first 7 ingredients, stirring well.

2. To prepare salad, combine lettuce and remaining ingredients in a large bowl. Drizzle dressing over salad; toss gently to coat. Serve immediately.

"If you can dream it, you can Achieve it!"

Made in the USA
Middletown, DE
05 January 2015